Summ

Why We Sleep

Unlocking the Power of Sleep and Dreams

BY

Matthew Walker, PhD

Table of Contents

Executive Summary

"I'd rather watch this TV show than sleep right now." You say as you comfortably settle in your bed at 1:20 AM with your laptop in front of you while you sip on a mug of your favorite cappuccino. You snuggle in the warm bed, with the heaters turned on. The rest of the world is snoozing in the peaceful arms of deep slumber. Your gaze flicks to the clock striking 2:00 AM. You mentally calculate that you still have five hours before you will have to get ready for work. Your eyes droop a little, but sleep is nowhere close to your mind as you are engrossed in the show.

Does this situation seem familiar to you? I'm sure it does. Every now and then, we ignore our sleep for something else. The blue light from your laptop, caffeine and even the heaters could be harming your ability to sleep.

If this intrigues you, this book is written for you.

It is not the opportunity to sleep that we lack. Rather, it's the lack of will to sleep. You might be wondering why this is so. We all have a general idea of the tiring day that awaits us after pulling an all-nighter. However, most of us don't realize the dire consequences that go beyond the next day.

Lack of sleep can have many negative effects on your physical and mental health. Furthermore, lack of sleep doesn't just affect you as an individual. Its effects extend to the workplace, organizations as well as the entire society.

In this book, we will explore everything you need to know about sleep. You will learn about its benefits to your body and mind. You will also learn about the effects of sleep deprivation. We will talk about sleeping pills and all the myths that revolve around them. We will also explore the realm of dreams.

So, this book is aimed at giving you the much-needed awareness about sleep. After you have gotten the basic knowledge about sleep, we will also discuss actionable advice to help you sleep better. The best thing about this book is that it won't tell you to lock away everything that harms your sleep. Rather, we will discuss how to sleep better while staying within our limits.

Chapter 1 -
What Is Sleep?

Key Knowledge Pointers

- Chronic sleep deprivation can have many ill effects on mental and physical health.

- Sleep plays a more vital role than even exercise and a balanced diet.

- It is only sleep that can reset our minds.

Two-thirds of adults fail to get eight hours of sleep each night. Sleeping for less than six to seven hours can have negative effects on our physical and mental well-being.

Lack of sleep can negatively affect your immunity and leave you prone to infections. Ignoring your sleep can also increase the risk of cancer by two-folds and leave you susceptible to Alzheimer's. Imagine that!

Furthermore, many individuals who don't get adequate sleep can become pre-diabetic and also carve their way towards many heart diseases.

The benefits of sleep are not limited to physical health only. Lack of sleep can also lead to major psychiatric illnesses including depression, anxiety, and increased suicide rates.

A disruption in your sleep routine can leave dire consequences on your overall lifestyle as well. For example, sleeping less will increase your appetite. So, dieting can only be a dream for those who don't sleep well. Even if you try to diet, you will lose lean body mass instead of fat.

Furthermore, a lack of sleep leads to a shorter life span. Not only will it decrease the number of years you will live, but it will also worsen the quality of your life.

World Health Organization has declared that sleep deprivation is prevalent in all developed countries. The industrialized nations suffer from many physical and mental diseases owing to a lack of good sleep.

So, sleep is the best 'pill' doctors can give for anything. However, this does not mean that doctors should prescribe sleeping pills. They have even worse effects on health as we will discuss later.

Moreover, in two circumstances a deterioration of sleep can even go as far as killing you. First, there is a rare genetic disorder in which the individual begins with insomnia, and progresses to no sleep at all before he dies in the next twelve to eighteen months. This disorder shows that a complete lack of sleep can indeed kill you. Second, drowsy driving is known to cause accidents more than drunk driving.

No one gives sleep its due importance because it has never been addressed adequately. Many greater scientists including Sigmund Freud, Francis Crick, Quintilian have tried to unravel sleep without any success.

Even from an evolutionary perspective, spending one-third of your life sleeping may seem to be stupid. You are not reproducing, gathering food, or protecting your offspring. So, it seems that it is evolution's mistake that sleep still exists.

However, the fact that sleep exists despite its apparent uselessness means that its pros outweigh the cons. So, sleep performs many complex functions for our brains, bodies, and daily functioning.

It is all thanks to sleep that we can learn, memorize, and think. Sleep enriches our emotional functioning as well.

Dreams while sleeping are also an essential part of our wellbeing. It creates a "virtual reality space" where our brain melds information, improves our creativity, and helps to deal with painful memories.

Sleep also improves the functions of our immune system and helps the body fight infections and germs. It improves our metabolic state and creates a balance between insulin and glucose.

Furthermore, sleep regulates our appetite and helps to maintain healthy body weight. A good night's sleep also flourishes the microbiome living in our gut.

Sleeping well also means that you will have better heart health, normal blood pressure and lower risk of cardiovascular diseases.

Many people are unaware that sleep plays a more vital role than even exercise and a balanced diet. So, the ill-effects of ignoring sleep are greater than ignoring diet and exercise.

Moreover, no other medically induced or natural state can have the same health benefits as sleeping naturally. Sleep is the single most effective thing that can "reset" our mind and physical well-being.

This summary book is written to provide accurate information about sleep and why it is so vital.

Chapter 2 -
Coffee, Jet lag & Natural Sleep Inducers

Key Knowledge Pointers

- There are two forces that decide your sleeping pattern. The circadian rhythm and sleep pressure.

- Everyone has a different circadian rhythm that is approximately twenty-four hours, with or without light.

- Melatonin is not an effective sleeping pill.

- Frequent jet lag can have many ill effects on one's mental and physical health.

- Caffeine is an addictive psychoactive stimulant that can "artificially mute" the effect of adenosine, making you feel alert.

Circadian Rhythm

There are two main factors that decide your sleep-wake pattern. The first factor is the internal twenty-four-hour clock. This internal clock creates a rhythm that decides when you are alert and when you are tired.

The second factor is a chemical that builds "sleep pressure." The longer you are awake, the more this chemical accumulates in your brain, and the more tired you will feel.

These two factors balance your cycle and determine your sleep-wake routine. This chemical also determines the quality of your sleep.

Every living creature has a circadian rhythm. Circa means 'around' and dian refers to 'day.' This clock in our brain sends signals to the rest of the organs as well. It controls other patterns like your body temperature, emotions, secretion of hormones, metabolic rate, eating timings, and even the amount of urine you produce.

For example, the time of the day determines the probability of winning an Olympic record. Even the timings of birth and deaths relate to the circadian rhythm.

In 1729, Jean-Jacques d'Ortous de Mairan stopped time for the plant Mimosa pudica that Charles Darwin called "sleeping leaves." This plant's leaves would open like an umbrella during day time and collapse at night time.

Many people believed that this rhythmic opening and closing were triggered by daylight and its absence.

To test this hypothesis, De Mairan put the plant in a sealed box for the next day. The box was completely dark. De Mairan observed that the plants behaved the same even in the complete absence of sunlight.

This meant that the plant could track time without any external cues such as daylight. So, the plant didn't just have a circadian rhythm. They had an "endogenous" or self-generated circadian rhythm.

It took another two centuries to prove that humans also possess a self-generated circadian rhythm.

In 1938, an experiment by Professor Nathaniel Kleitman and his assistant Bruce Richardson lead to more ground-breaking discoveries. Both experimenters took a trip to the Mammoth Cave in Kentucky where no sunlight can penetrate. They stayed there for thirty-two days with a supply of food and water along with some measuring devices to record their sleep-wake cycles.

Despite being in complete darkness, they had regular and predictable sleeping patterns. They would sleep for about nine hours and stay awake for fifteen. This proved a few things. First, humans don't need sunlight to have a regular circadian rhythm. Surprisingly, the circadian rhythm is around twenty-four hours long even in the absence of daylight. This led to a new way of defining the circadian rhythm. Their cycles were approximately twenty-four hours long. So, the length of the rhythm is not precisely one day.

After this experiment, the duration has been determined to be around twenty-four hours and fifteen minutes.

However, sunlight does help to reset our internal clock if it becomes more imprecise. This is because sunlight is the most reliable signal that repeats at designated times every day.

There are many external signals, termed as "zeitgeber" from German "time giver," that our brain uses to reset our biological clock whenever it needs to. Many cues such as routinely eating, exercising, temperature fluctuations and even timed social interaction to serve to help our biological timepiece stick to a twenty-four hours duration. The most obvious example of this is that blind people keep their circadian rhythm around the twenty-four hours mark just like everyone else.

So, daylight serves as the main zeitgeber, but other external cues also help to set the biological clock.

The biological clock is known as the suprachiasmatic nucleus. Supra means above and chiasm means a crossing point. So, the suprachiasmatic nucleus lies just above the crossing point of the optic nerves. So, the light signals from our eyes can help to reset any time inaccuracy in the twenty-four-hour cycle.

It is composed of 20,000 cells but takes very little space. This suprachiasmatic nucleus controls a variety of rhythmic patterns including the core temperature. The body temperature begins to rise during the day, peaks in the late afternoon, drops to its lowest point two hours before sleep onset, and then begins to rise again.

This "pre-programmed" rhythm will repeat every twenty-four hours whether you sleep or not. So, your circadian rhythm controls your sleep-wake cycle.

Everyone has a different rhythm

The high and low points of any rhythmic pattern are different for everyone. You may be a morning person like 40% of the population, evening person like the 30%, or fall somewhere in between like the rest of the 30% of the population. This is known as the chronotype.

The prefrontal cortex of the brain controls higher-level functioning and reasoning. So, if an evening person wakes up too early, their prefrontal cortex doesn't work as well.

Your chronotype is not a choice. It is determined by your DNA makeup and genetics.

People treat evening people unfairly by deeming them as lazy. Also, the workplace runs during the morning. This gives an edge to the morning people as they are well-slept and fresher than the evening people.

So, evening folks are known to be inclined toward being sleep-deprived, depressed, anxious, diabetic, and even more prone to cancer, heart issues, and stroke.

So, just like physical differences such as blindness matter, society needs to facilitate and provide for evening people too.

This genetic variation in sleeping patterns have an evolutionary advantage. Due to this variability, everyone in a group is not sleeping for eight hours straight. Rather, half of the people are sleeping while the other half are awake. The entire group is sleeping at the same time for only a few hours rather than eight hours. This contributes to protecting the group and not leaving everyone vulnerable.

Melatonin

How does the suprachiasmatic nucleus talk to the body? It sends out a hormone known as melatonin from the pineal gland.

Melatonin determines the time you will sleep. Contrary to the common perception, melatonin doesn't aid you in sleeping. So, apart from the placebo effect, over-the-counter melatonin is not a useful sleeping pill.

The brain releases melatonin a few hours after dusk and it drops down around the time of dawn. When the melatonin secretion decreases and sunlight penetrates your closed eyelids, it's time to wake up naturally.

Jet Lag

When we travel to a new time zone faster than our brain can adapt to the change, you experience jet lag. You feel drowsy during the day time of the new time zone because your body thinks that it is night time.

You slowly get used to the change due to external cues. For each day you are in a different place, your clock will readjust by one hour.

Jet lag is not just uncomfortable as you can't fall asleep at the right time. It has many negative health effects. First, the parts of the brain relating to learning and memory physically shrink. Secondly, short term memory is affected. Pilots and other jet crews are more prone to cancer and type 2 diabetes.

A way of fighting with jet lag is melatonin. It helps to fool the brain into thinking that it is time to sleep. However, melatonin does not help you fall asleep quicker.

Sleep Pressure

When the chemical adenosine builds up in our brain, we experience a desire to sleep. This urge is known as sleep pressure.

The greater the amount of adenosine, the more powerful the urge to go to sleep will be.

Most people experience sleep pressure after 12 to 16 hours of being awake.

Caffeine

Caffeine is an addictive psychoactive stimulant that can "artificially mute" the effect of adenosine, making you feel alert. Caffeine works by blocking the adenosine receptors in the brain.

Caffeine begins to kick in action after half an hour of intake. It has a half-life of 5-7 hours. So, the cup of espresso you took after lunch can stop you from falling asleep at night.

An enzyme from the liver breaks down caffeine and removes it from your body. Our sensitivity to caffeine is determined by our genetics. Furthermore, as you age, you become more sensitive to the effects of caffeine.

After the liver has removed all the caffeine from your body, you may experience a "caffeine crash." You are hit with a strong urge to sleep due to the adenosine built up in your system.

The Two Forces

As I explained earlier, the two forces that determine your sleep pattern are the suprachiasmatic nucleus's melatonin and adenosine's sleep pressure. These two forces are separate and don't work together to regulate your sleep. They may be aligned but don't work in conjunction with each other.

When the low level of adenosine is aligned with the activating output of the suprachiasmatic nucleus, you will be wide awake. Similarly, when there is a low activity level due to a low circadian rhythm aligned with strong sleep pressure, you will feel a powerful urge to sleep.

You wake up naturally after you have slept for eight to nine hours, the body has removed the adenosine and the circadian rhythm has picked up.

 Both these processes work independently. You will notice this when you pull an all-nighter. Despite being up the previous night, you may feel energetic and alert. This is due to your circadian activity peaking despite the build-up of adenosine and sleep pressure.

Adequate Sleep

Do you need caffeine before noon?

Do you feel sleepy before 12 PM after waking up in the morning?

If the answer to both questions is yes, then you are not getting adequate or quality sleep.

Prolonged sleep deprivation can cause a host of health issues as discussed in Chapter 1.

Chapter 3 -
How We Actually Sleep

Key Knowledge Pointers

- There are many cues that help you identify when someone else is asleep and not dead or in a coma.

- There are two types of sleep: low-frequency NREM sleep and high-frequency REM sleep.

- The waking state is for "reception," NREM sleep for "reflection," and REM sleep for "integration."

Identifying Sleep

There are many cues that tell you that someone is sleeping.

1. The person's position is a tell-tale sign that they're sleeping.
2. The muscles are relaxed and the body is slouched.
3. The person doesn't communicate in any way.
4. Sleep is reversible; the person will wake up due to noise
5. Sleep has a reliable pattern.

How do you know that you slept?

Often, we assess the quality and timing of our own sleep. So, how does anyone himself know that there were asleep?

1. We lose touch with our surroundings

2. Our sense of time is distorted.

The thalamus is the sensory gateway in our brain. When we are sleeping, we have a "sensory blackout." This is because the thalamus blocks the sensory stimuli from reaching the cortices of the brain. So, even though you are hearing, your brain doesn't perceive and interpret those sound waves.

Secondly, our brain experiences a distorted time. Often, we experience time dilation. The time zone in our dreams is longer than it really is. This is because the experiences are being "replayed" at a slower speed.

The two types of sleep

Scientifically, sleep is accessed by the following.

1. Brainwave activity
2. Eye movement
3. Muscle tone

These three stimuli are collectively known as PSG or polysomnography. It is a graph of numerous signals (poly) that occur during sleep (Somnus).

Professor Kleitman and his student Eugene Aserinsky found the two different types of sleep: NREM or non-rapid eye movement, and REM or rapid eye movement.

REM sleep has brain waves just like we are awake. In this phase, we dream.

NREM sleep is divided into four stages termed as stages 1 to 4.

The Sleep Cycle

Each sleep cycle is of ninety minutes. Our sleep is NREM sleep in the first half of the night. The second half consists of REM sleep. Each phase is repeatable but asymmetric.

NREM sleep is designed to remove the neural connections that are not needed. On the other hand, REM sleep works to strengthen the remaining connections. So, in the first half of the night that is dominated by NREM sleep focuses on removing the unnecessary parts of our neural connections with a little fine-tuning from the REM sleep. After the connections have been built in the first half, the second half works to "enhance" and "detail" those neural connections with REM sleep.

So, if you sleep for six hours instead of eight, you will be losing a cycle of your sleep. Whether you lose the REM or NREM part, you will suffer from ill effects on your mental and physical health.

Types of Brainwaves

Before you go to bed, your brain is in an active state. It produces fast frequency waves. These waves don't have a clear pattern or rhythm. These waves are "chaotic" because of the number of stimuli the brain must interpret from each of the senses (sight, sound, smell, taste, emotions).

After you drift into a sleepy state, you first cross the shallow stages of NREM sleep. Then, you are plunged into the deeper stages 3 and 4 of NREM sleep. These stages are characterized by slow waves that are about tenfold slower than the brain waves while you are awake.

So, the slow-wave NREM is more reliable and predictable.

While you are in deep sleep, you will exhibit a new peak of activity known as the sleep spindle. These sleep spindles protect you from external sounds so that your sleep is not disturbed.

These deep waves originate from the center of the frontal lobes. Instead of traveling in circles, these waves will travel in one direction only. These low-frequency waves serve as the default mode that allows the cortex to "relax" as the thalamus blocks the transfer of all stimuli from the environment. This state of deep sleep has many benefits for our physical and mental health. For example, these slow waves during NREM sleep help to consolidate your memories.

Also, the slow NREM sleep waves help to communicate with distant regions of the brain and store memories.

On the other hand, the fast-frequency brain activity during REM sleep resembles that of the waking state. It is nearly impossible to differentiate between the two patterns of brain waves.

The only way to tell the difference is by looking at the muscle tone. During REM sleep, the muscles lose their tension and become limp. The body is almost "paralyzed." The electrodes attached to the body show "atonia" or an absence of tone. This is done by a signal from your brain stem to the spinal cord. So, your arms and legs are completely disabled.

During REM sleep, our brain gives out many motor signals. So, a paralysis-like state is essential during REM sleep. Otherwise, we would act out on all the bizarre fictional movements from our dreams. So, Mother Nature has ensured that we can dream safely by paralyzing our bodies.

Also, recent studies have found that the brain is 30% more active during REM sleep as compared to when we are awake. So, REM sleep is known as paradoxical sleep.

Moreover, the thalamus gate is also open during REM sleep. The only difference is that it is not open to external stimuli. Rather, the sensory gate lets in sensations from past experiences and memories to be exchanged in the brain. So, everything plays out at a slower speed and REM sleep strengthens the neural connections.

So, the waking state is for the "reception" of information as you receive it from the environment around you.

You can think of NREM sleep as the "reflection" of information as the brain strengthens the memories.

The REM sleep serves the "integration" purpose. It establishes connections between the experiences and remodels them.

Chapter 4 -
The Sleep of Different Species

Key Knowledge Pointers

- Sleep is an unnegotiable, unifying feature across the entire animal kingdom.

- Sleep is varied in terms of the amount, form (half brain vs whole brain), pattern (monophasic, biphasic, and polyphasic).

The History of Sleep

To study the history of sleep, we must go back to the evolutionary tree.

Every animal species including the insect's phyla, fish, sharks, amphibians, frogs, reptiles, turtles, chameleons, parrots, kangaroos, polar bears, bats sleeps. Invertebrate species like the mollusks and echinoderms also had their share of sleep.

The worms dated back to the Cambrian explosion also snoozed off. So, sleep is at least 500 million years old. Even dinosaurs and diplodocuses slept in their time.

So, sleep is not only quite old, but it is also universal. Even unicellular organisms went into a sleep-like state.

So, why did sleep evolve? Was it meant to fix the things that had become "upset" while the organism was awake?

Or was it that sleep evolved first, and from sleep-wakefulness came into being?

Whatever the case, one thing we know for sure is that that sleep is one of the earliest forms of life known to this planet. It is a uniting feature of the different phyla in the animal kingdom.

So, how is the sleep of other species different from our sleep?

Duration

The duration of sleep is different across the animal kingdom.

Elephants sleep for four hours, almost half the time as humans. On the other hand, lions sleep for fifteen hours and bats for nineteen hours.

Sleep doesn't follow a regular pattern as you would expect from the phylum tree. For instance, squirrels sleep for 15.8 hours while degu sleep for 7.7 hours. Despite the difference in sleep duration, both these organisms are part of the same family. On the other hand, the guinea pig and baboon belong to different phylogenetic orders but sleep for an equal duration: 9.4 hours.

So, why is the duration so different even within the same phylogenetic family?

The complexity and size of the nervous system is a good reason. So, as the size of the brain functions become complex, the need for sleep increases.

However, we need to give due importance to the quality of the sleep. So, the species that have a better quality of sleep may need lesser time. This may be logical but, it is not so. Those animals that have a higher quality sleep often tend to sleep more. Furthermore, the quality of sleep cannot be measured operationally.

Scientists believe that the duration of sleep is based on several factors. For example, the metabolic rate, type of nervous system, animal's predatory nature and dietary type determine the quantity and quality of sleep. So, the evolutionary path of sleep is shaped by many forces.

Despite such predictions, there are many outliers. For example, giraffes sleep for only four to five hours.

Composition of Sleep

The second difference in sleep among species is composition. Many species do not experience all the stages of sleep like humans do.

One thing to note is that all species go through NREM sleep. Birds and mammals experience REM sleep. Insects, fish, and most reptiles do not go through REM stages at all.

So, NREM stages are the pioneer. REM sleep emerged much later in the evolutionary tree. It seems that REM sleep evolved to make sleep deeper and support the NREM stages.

However, dolphins and whales don't abide by the other mammal's sleeping pattern. They don't experience the REM phase at all.

A possible explanation for this could be that REM sleep paralyzes the organism's muscles, making it immobile. If aquatic mammals become immobile, they would not be able to keep afloat and drown while they are sleeping.

This explanation is also backed up by pinnipeds such as fur seals. They spend their time on both the land and sea. On land, they experience both REM and NREM sleep. In the ocean, they stop having REM sleep. So, REM sleep is not feasible for aquatic mammals.

Even if they have a different form of REM sleep, it is not detected yet as their brain waves are difficult to measure.

Furthermore, REM sleep evolved twice in the evolutionary tree. It emerged in the mammals and birds separately. So, birds and mammals probably faced similar environmental pressures that carved the way for REM sleep. This shows the importance of REM sleep.

In warm-blooded mammals and birds, REM sleep has many benefits from improved heart health and temperature regulation to creativity, memory association, and emotional IQ.

A fundamental question is what type of sleep do we need more?

To test this, many experiments have been performed. All of them come to the following conclusions.

First, the recovery night for sleep-deprived individuals is always longer than the normal duration of sleep. Second, lack of NREM sleep rebounds harder. So, on the first recovery night, your brain will spend more time in NREM sleep to respond to the debt. However, on the second, third and fourth nights after sleep deprivation, the brain will focus on REM sleep.

This shows that both types of sleep are vital. The brain first tries to pay the debt for NREM sleep and then for REM sleep.

One thing you must know is that you can never get the get back all the sleep you lost. So, what's lost is lost.

The Way We Sleep

The third remarkable difference between sleep across species is the way of sleeping.

For example, dolphins and whales have only NREM sleep that is "unihemispheric." This means that they sleep with half a brain at a time. The other half of the brain stays awake to ward off any threats and maintain movement in the water. Even though both the cerebral hemispheres are separated by a thin band of fibers, it is possible that one half of the brain is bathed in slow, rhythmic brain waves and the other half with fast, frantic brain activity.

Even with half of the brain active at a time, dolphins exhibit an excellent level of communication. When the dolphin is awake, it can use both of its hemispheres at the same time. However, when it needs to sleep it must uncouple.

So, it is obvious that sleep has far greater benefits than disadvantages that Mother Nature did not eradicate sleep from evolution. So, there's no option to not sleep.

Apart from aquatic animals, birds also exhibit this split-shift system of sleep. It allows them to keep an eye out for predators and other threats.

Humans don't have this ability of sleeping. However, recent studies show that we do have a mild version of this sleep. The brain waves during NREM sleep will be different for someone sleeping at their home and when they sleep in a new place like a sleep lab or hotel. The latter environments are unfamiliar and may pose a threat. So, half of the brain has adapted to sleep lighter than the other half. As the individual gets used to the new place, the activity in both halves of the brain becomes similar. So, now you know why you sleep lightly on the first night in a hotel.

However, in the REM phase, the brain waves in both halves of the brain are the same. So, even in a new environment, it is not possible to sleep lightly with one half of the brain. This is the same in every species including birds and the aquatic mammals who have REM sleep.

Sleep Patterns

When an organism is in an extreme situation, it will sleep much lesser than normal. For example, in a famine, the organism will give more importance to food than to sleep. The brain is fooled into believing that if they sleep, they won't get food.

For example, if you starve a fly, it will sleep lesser.

This sleep pattern is also prevalent in killer whales. They give birth to a calf away from the other members. When the killer whale and calf must travel back to swim back, both the calf and mother don't sleep even though a newborn needs a lot of sleep after the first few days after birth.

This pattern of sleep deprivation without any harm is also seen in birds during migration across an ocean due to climate changes. The birds fly more than normal and they should need more sleep to rest. However, they can easily forgo their sleep in such a situation without any adverse effects. Birds have also evolved an excellent mechanism of sleeping for only a few seconds to refresh their energy.

The US military is interested in such patterns of deliberate sleep deprivation without any ill effects on health. Imagine having a twenty-four-hour soldier!

Monophasic and Biphasic Sleep

In most industrialized countries, humans sleep in a monophasic pattern. They have a total of seven hours of sleep during the night.

In pre-industrialized countries, you will notice that people have a biphasic pattern – that is, they sleep for a long period at night followed by a thirty to sixty-minute nap in the afternoon.

Such a biphasic sleep pattern is more prevalent during the hot summer season.

The practice of biphasic sleep emerged to cater to the mid-afternoon dip in alertness. This is known as a post-prandial alertness dip. It is a normal part innate in everyone. It seems that Mother Nature has created this dip to try to make up for the lost sleep.

So, there is genetic and biological evidence of biphasic sleep. Forgoing this sleep pattern has many negative effects on health.

Harvard University's School of Public Health conducted a study on more than 23,000 Greek adults to analyse the effects of shifting from a biphasic to a monophasic pattern.

It contributes to a 37% increase in the risk of death due to cardiovascular disease, especially among working men.

Tree to Ground

Humans are special in many domains including sleep.

First, the total amount of time we spend sleeping is different than apes such as chimpanzees and gorillas. We sleep for eight hours while they sleep for ten to fifteen hours.

20 to 25% of our sleep is dedicated to REM sleep, while only 9% of their sleep is REM sleep.

Primates used to sleep on trees and nests while we are "terrestrial sleepers." Sleeping in trees seemed to contribute to survival in terms of safety from night predators. However, sleeping thirty feet up in the air can be dangerous too. Balancing the body on a tree branch, especially during REM sleep can be difficult.

So, Homo erectus, our predecessor started sleeping on the ground. They would light a fire to keep away the predators at night. Sleeping on the ground increased the portion of REM sleep.

REM sleep contributed to our emotional IQ, cognitive intelligence, creativity, and degree of social complexity. So, we can say that we are special thanks to the evolution of REM sleep.

Chapter 5 -
Sleep Changes During Our Life

Key Knowledge Pointers

- In fetuses, six hours are allocated for NREM sleep, six for REM, and the remaining twelve hours are in an intermediary type of sleep. In the third trimester, the infant starts to spend about two to three hours awake.

- Young children and infants show a pattern of polyphasic sleep in contrast to their parents' monophasic pattern.

- There is a rise in the quality and intensity of deep sleep as the child must build more connections. During adolescence, NREM sleep increases to build cognitive skills and reasoning. So, deep sleep is a vital driving force of brain maturation.

- Senior adults need as much sleep as they needed in midlife but it decreases due to the following three factors: reduced quantity/quality, reduced sleep efficiency and disrupted timing.

Neonates and Newborns' Sleep

Before birth, the baby will just sleep in the mother's womb. The kick mothers feel is not the baby's response to anything; it is due to the bursts of brain activity during REM sleep.

You might be thinking that the body should be paralyzed during REM sleep. This isn't the case with the fetus. The muscle-inhibiting mechanism is not in place yet.

At this stage, the infant sleeps a lot. During the twenty-four hours, six hours are allocated for NREM sleep, six for REM, and the remaining twelve hours are in an intermediary type of sleep. In the third trimester, the infant starts to spend about two to three hours awake.

In the last two weeks of pregnancy, the infant spends time in REM sleep for almost nine hours. In the last week of pregnancy, the fetus spends twelve hours in REM sleep. However, the fetus doesn't actually fully sleep in this REM sleep as the brain has not fully matured yet.

The increase in REM sleep in the second and third trimesters coincides with the time of brain development and maturation. In this period, synaptogenesis takes place.

If the mother's intake of alcohol blocks REM sleep, brain development is halted. Newborns of heavy-drinking mothers also show a decreased quality and quantity of REM sleep. There is a 200% reduction in the measure of brain waves associated with REM sleep.

Alcohol also depressed the breathing rate during REM sleep from 381 per hour to just 4 per hour.

Feeding mothers who consume alcohol affect the infant's REM sleep as well. The newborn suffers from a 20 to 30% decrease in REM sleep. The baby's sleep is also fragmented.

During the first few months, REM sleep is essential for the baby's development. Every hour counts towards development. So, disruption of REM sleep in fetuses or neonates can distort brain development significantly, leaving the child prone to many mental disorders.

REM sleep deficiency has is also linked to ASD or autism spectrum disorder. Autism relates to abnormal synaptogenesis. It results in a weaker circadian rhythm and less melatonin. So, autistic children suffer a 30 to 50% decrease in their REM sleep duration as compared to normal children who don't have autism. However, we can't claim that autism and REM sleep deficit are the main causes for each other.

Sleep in Childhood

Young children and infants show a pattern of polyphasic sleep in contrast to their parents' monophasic pattern.

This is because the child's suprachiasmatic nucleus is not developed fully. It is by the age of three to four months before the child's circadian rhythm improves a little due to the repeating signals such as daylight, feeding, and temperature changes.

By the first year, the child will move towards short naps during the day. By four years, the circadian rhythm improves more. The child transitions from polyphasic sleep to biphasic sleep. It is only in late childhood when the child begins to show a pattern of monophasic sleep.

The total duration of sleep decreases after birth. However, the ratio of time in NREM and REM doesn't decline in the same pattern.

A six-month baby sleeps for an average of 14 hours with an equal time spent in NREM and REM stages. A five-year-old child sleeps for a total of 11 hours with a 70:30 ratio of NREM and REM sleep.

So, the duration of REM sleep decreases and the amount of NREM sleep increases during childhood.

Sleep in Adolescents

NREM sleep increases after birth because it helps to remodel and prune the neural connections and pathways formed by REM sleep. The brain reshapes and refines the original structure formed by REM sleep.

Irwin Feinberg, a pioneer of sleep research, conducted extensive studies in adolescents.

During middle and late childhood, he observed that there is a moderate amount of deep sleep. There is a rise in the quality and intensity of deep sleep as the child must build more connections. During adolescence, NREM sleep increases to build cognitive skills and reasoning. So, deep sleep is one of the most vital driving forces of brain maturation.

If deep sleep is disturbed by caffeine or sleep deprivation, maturation is also affected and this carves the way for many mental illnesses such as ADHD, depression, bipolar disorder, schizophrenia, etc.

If the refinement of the neural connection is abnormal especially in the frontal lobe which controls higher-level thinking, the adolescent is set on a pathway of schizophrenia.

Adolescents struggle to get the recommended amount of sleep as their circadian rhythm is set at a forward schedule than their parents. They want to sleep late at night and then wake up later as well. Due to early school times, they are forced to wake up early. Also, teenagers need more sleep than adults. When these two add up, the adolescent ends up becoming sleep deprived.

The reason that biology has set teenagers' circadian rhythm ahead is so that they can enjoy some hours of independence.

Midlife and Old Age

Senior adults need as much sleep as they needed in midlife but it decreases due to the following three factors.

1. Reduced quantity/quality
2. Reduced sleep efficiency
3. Disrupted timing

Sleep can get fragmented, thus losing the quantity and quality. The older adults' sleep gets interrupted due to medications, diseases and a weakened bladder.

This reduces the efficiency of sleep – the time spent sleeping while you were in bed. Good sleep efficiency is above 90%. In the eighties, the sleep efficiency reduces below 70 to 80% -- more than one and a half hours is spent awake while in bed.

This has many negative effects on physical health as well as cognitive functioning. They will report lesser energy, depression, and forgetfulness.

The third change is due to an altered circadian rhythm that has moved to an earlier time. Melatonin will be secreted in the late evening. As the older adult will take a nap, the adenosine and sleep pressure will decrease. This will keep them awake in the night. In the morning, as the circadian rhythm rises, the older adult will wake up early. When these two aspects add up, older adults become sleep deprived.

An effective solution to this is taking melatonin pills in the late evening and daylight exposure in the late afternoon instead of the morning.

You might be thinking why there is a loss of quantity and quality of sleep in the first place.

This is because the structures that produce sleep start to deteriorate. This is known as atrophy of neurons. So, older individuals suffer from a 70% deficit in deep sleep with accompanying effects on memory and cognition.

Chapter 6 -
The Wonders of Sleep

Key Knowledge Pointers

- Sleep is a medicine that can offer many cures.

- All types and stages of sleep are equally important.

- Sleep has many functions.

- After sleeping for the night, the individual would retrieve the memory from the neocortex instead of the hippocampus.

Sleep is a medicine that can offer many cures. What's astounding is that this medicine offers preventions as well. Furthermore, it is free.

Due to a lack of awareness, we tend to ignore the benefits of sleep.

Sleep for the Brain

When you sleep, you just don't sleep. In other words, sleep is much more than just sleep as we know it. As we established in the previous chapters, sleep is a state of consciousness where our brain is very active and transitions through different stages.

36

Also, it is essential to remember that all types and stages of sleep are equally important.

Sleep has many functions. For example, it serves to improve your memory. So, the memory pills you need to enhance your retention of facts is none other than sleep.

It not only helps in the retention of previous information, but it also helps to create new memories.

Sleep the Night Before

For fact-based learning, such as cramming for an exam or remembering someone's email address, the hippocampus in your brain will aid you. It is the region of the brain that helps to store information for a short period of time.

If your hippocampus is overflowed with information, you will not be able to add more information to it or it will start to "overwrite." This is known as interference forgetting.

However, the good news is that sleep helps to empty the hippocampus. When we sleep, the information is shifted from the hippocampus to a permanent reservoir in our brain. This refreshes the capacity of the hippocampus and allows for new learning.

This was tested in a study. Two groups of adults were randomly selected. There were both taught some facts. Then, one group could take a short nap while the other wasn't.

Later, on the same day, both the groups went through another round of intensive learning. As expected, the group that took a nap memorized the facts better. An astounding 20%

improvement was noticed in their ability to learn new facts as compared to the no-nap group.

So, it can be established that sleep empties up room for new information as the brain transfer information. This refreshment was noticed in the lighter stage known as stage 2 of NREM sleep where sleep spindles are released. It was evident that the number of sleep spindles was related to the replenishment of learning ability.

The transfer of information from the short-term reservoir, hippocampus, to the long-term location, cortex, is electrical in nature.

This finding also relates to the deficit in learning capacity related to aging. Older adults experience fewer number of spindles during their sleep. This correlates with their decreased ability to cram facts and retain them.

Another important thing that most people don't know is that NREM sleep spindles occur in the late-morning hours. So, those who sleep for six hours or lesser will experience the lesser benefit of sleep in terms of the replenishment it offers.

Sleep the Night After

Another benefit of sleeping is the one that comes after learning. This is known as the consolidation of memory.

The time we spent sleeping after learning helps to consolidate the newly learning facts and prevents forgetting. Studies have found this to be true by at least 20 to 40% better retention. This has evolutionary advantages too as it helps in the survival of the fittest.

In the 1950s, effort was made to understand how sleep helps to consolidate facts. It was established that the NREM stage of sleep helps to solidify information.

In the early 2000s, many studies were done for this. All of them had the same finding: the more the NREM sleep at night, the more the individual could remember information the next day.

So, it is even possible to predict how well you will remember facts based on your NREM sleep quality.

Using MRI scans, researchers have investigated the location of memories before and after. It was found that the memories had been moved to a physically different location. After sleeping for the night, the individual would retrieve the memory from the neocortex instead of the hippocampus.

So, the slow brainwaves during NREM sleep transferred the memories from the short-term storage to the long-term one. This empties the short-term storage and also solidifies previous memories.

Also, sleep helps to retrieve the memories that you think you've forgotten. The brain repairs those memories during sleep so that you can have access to them the next day.

It is also possible to experimentally enhance the benefits of sleep for memory:

1. Stimulation
2. Targeted memory activation

Stimulation is done by inserting small amounts of voltage to the brain during NREM sleep to enhance the deep brainwaves.

Researchers doubled the number of facts retained by doing this.

Another method used quiet auditory tones to stimulate sleep resulting in a 40% memory improvement.

However, if you try this yourself, it could result in impairing the quality of your sleep among other issues.

Another finding was made that rocking or swaying the bed boosted the quality of brain waves and thus sleep spindles. So, rocking an infant back and forth has more health benefits than we realize.

The second thing was targeted memory activation. This is like selecting only the memories you want and deleting the unwanted ones.

Researchers did this by auditory-tagging images while the participants were sleeping. This helped the brain to discriminate between the memories and selecting the ones that were tagged.

Imagine the ability to rewrite your life!

Sleeping to Forget

We think that forgetting is bad, but it is actually not. In fact, it's just as important as remembering.

Simply put, it is not possible to remember new facts without forgetting the unnecessary information. For example, remembering information such as who you saw on the way to work is not really useful. So, our brain works to forget such information.

Francis Crick also worked to discover the astounding capabilities of sleep. He thought that REM sleep worked to remove the unwanted parts of memory.

For example, research was conducted to find out the effects of naps on retention. If facts are tagged with a label that decides whether they should be remembered or not, sleeping will select the information that is tagged for remembering. However, this is not done during the REM stage as Crick predicted. The sleep spindles during NREM sleep work to dispose of the unnecessary parts of memory.

The information is actively transferred to the frontal lobe from the hippocampus.

Now, research is being conducted to use sleep to delete unwanted pieces of memory.

Sleeping for Other Memories

Sleeping also helps in consolidating the routines associated with "muscle memory." For example, sleeping can help to improve a pianist's skills. So, practice along with sleep makes perfect.

It also helps to improve the accuracy of the skills. This improvement occurs during stage 2 of NREM sleep, especially during the last two hours of sleep. Such memories are saved in the motor cortex of the brain.

This was also explored in athletes and the Olympics. Daytime naps improve energy levels and motor skills. Athletes who get less than eight hours of sleep suffer reduced muscle strength, oxygen saturation, and it also impairs the cardiovascular system and respiration. Also, lack of sleep increases the risk of injury.

Sleeping after the competition helps to improve physical recovery as well.

Sleep is also related to an improved level of creativity.

Chapter 7 -
Extreme Problems of Sleep Deprivation

Key Knowledge Pointers

- Sleep deprivation can lead to sleep while driving. It could be a microsleep or a longer duration.

- Sleep deprivation is the major cause of emotional irrationality and memory loss.

- Sleep deprivation and Alzheimer's disease are highly correlated.

Pay Attention

Insufficient sleep can lead to the most deadly and fatal events of your life. It disturbs the psychological functioning of your brain. You can be a culprit of sleep deprivation in two ways. For example, you can fall in deep sleep while driving, or sometimes you can fall into microsleep even if it's for a few seconds.

These few seconds are enough to drift your car and kill you. In the case of microsleep, your brain becomes blind to the real world and you will feel like all the perceptions of your brain are lost out.

This is not only thing that you face during sleep deprivation. Your performance level also suffers. For efficient cognitive performance, proper sleep is essential. The human brain needs more than seven hours of sleep, but if one does not have proper sleep for the length of 10 days it then leads to the dysfunction of the brain.

Can three full nights sleep be a recovery sleep? The answer is no! If your brain becomes dysfunctional, you cannot get the recovery sleep with three full days of consecutive sleep.

Can Naps Help for Sleep Deprivation?

There is no scientific basis to support the scenario of a nap. For the time being, you will feel like a nap increases your concentration level. However, it would not be beneficial for you psychologically. The functioning of the brain is very complex as it is involved in emotional stability, decision making, concentrating, remembering, and learning.

However, on the other hand, a rare number of individuals are found out who have their normal functioning of the brain even after 6 hours of sleep. No matter how much they work in a laboratory they just wake up after 6 hours of sleep without any reminder or alarm. This is due to their genetic makeup.

In addition, one can have a detailed explanation after studying genetic factors. A sub-variant gene called BHLHE41 is responsible for this.

Emotional Irrationality

Emotional irrationality is highly related to sleep deprivation. If you do not sleep well at night, it will change your mood and disturb you emotionally. Your brain will face chronic issues by not getting proper sleep. The emotional center of the brain is the striatum which is part of the amygdala. Sleep deprivation is also a major cause of aggression, irritability, bullying, and mood swings.

Other than this, the sleep deprivation is also a major reason of forgetting things earlier. This occurs due to the poor neuron connections between the brains. Proteins are the major source of the building blocks to have strong memories. It can also influence DNA, as per the recent studies. Sleep deprivation will prevent DNA from making your memory stronger and you will not be able to recall things.

Sleep and Alzheimer's Disease:

Sleep deprivation is highly linked to Alzheimer's disease. A decrease in NREM sleep can reduce the ability in memory in the same way like that of someone suffering from the Alzheimer's disease. For folks who are sleep deprived, they have a higher chance of developing the said disease. According to research, it is found out that all the patients with Alzheimer's disease have a clinical disorder, the most common form of which is insomnia.

Alzheimer disease is responsible for producing a harmful substance called beta-amyloid that later accumulates in the brain. In addition, this area of the brain is the frontal lobe where NREM is occurring. Due to massive accumulation of the substance, a person cannot have proper sleep time. This is how both are linked to each other where initial sleep deprivation increases the odds of developing the disease, then the disease itself manufacturing chemicals which impede the quality of sleep. A vicious cycle is thus born.

Chapter 8 -
Physiological Effects of Sleeping Less

Key Knowledge Pointers

- Sufficient sleep is the pillar of normal body functioning.

- Sleep deprivation does have a deep relationship with cardiovascular diseases and hypertension.

- It is the major cause of affecting the reproductive and developing immune system.

- Sleep deprivation is the major cause of obesity, and it affects cells, genes and DNA also.

Sleeping is considered the pillar of having good health. However, most folks do not have any idea how badly inadequate sleep can affect his or her health. Every part, every cell, and even every tissue of your body is affected if you are not having proper sleep. It can also alter the functioning of DNA that gives life and strength to your body. Many of the diseases that can lead to the death of a person including heart diseases, dementia, obesity, diabetes, and cancer can trace part of their cause to lack of sleep. Inadequate sleep can disturb the proper functioning of our cardiovascular system. Our metabolic, immune, and as well as reproductive systems are also at risk. It means that we are definitely affected by sleep deprivation.

Sleep Loss on the Cardiovascular and Reproductive system:

Inadequate sleep leads to fatal diseases, and according to research, it is found out that 45% of the population has a high risk of death due to decreased sleep. The chances of developing cardiovascular disease increase with age. At 45 years old, the risk of developing heart disease increases by 200% just due to the lack of sleep.

Blood pressure does not remain normal if you do not have enough sleep, then high blood pressure leads to heart problems. The systolic blood pressure in the heart does increase due to the decrease in sleep. In addition, this systolic pressure affects the physical fitness of a person as well.

The blood vessels known as coronary arteries feeding the heart do not work properly if one is sleep deprived. The coronary arteries tend to narrow and become constricted when sleep deprivation kicks in. This then creates problems for the heart as it becomes starved of vital oxygen supply, which then most often leads to the "massive coronary", a massive and most commonly fatal heart attack.

Atherosclerosis, or the shrinking and hardening of arterial walls via calcium deposits, are also most commonly exacerbated in folks who have sleeping periods of 6 hours or less. This once again places sleep deprived folk in higher danger of heart attacks, as narrowed and hardened arterial walls aren't exactly all good for the heart. Another major issue

48

caused by chronic sleep deprivation is the stress that it places on the sympathetic nervous system. This system is responsible for the marshalling of all of the body's innate resources, with which it will deploy in accordance to our normal human requirements, and also in response to any perceived threats. A lack of sleep is seen as a threat by the sympathetic nervous system, and hence it deploys the body's resources in an effort to address it. Think of it this way, lack of sleep is akin to a need for speed because you are perhaps driving somewhere urgently and hence you floor the accelerator of your vehicle. That flooring of the accelerator is the sympathetic nervous system's response. Now if you are constantly sleep deprived, that means the accelerator is constantly floored. Imagine how overheated and stressed the engine of the vehicle would be; and the same goes for your body.

This constant state of overdrive seen in the sympathetic nervous system then leads to high blood pressure and then to heart diseases. Cortisol, a stress hormone, is produced in larger quantities during stressful situations and when the body undergoes sleep deprivation. This hormone leads to hypertensive blood pressure and an increase in the rate of heartbeat.

As compared to this, proper sleep will keep the functioning of the sympathetic nervous system within its normal limits, thus taking care of your cardiovascular system. The communication of the brain with the body's regulation of other hormones does occur in a soothing way and hence major issues with blood pressure and coronary problems are mostly laid to rest.

Weight Gain and Obesity

It is obvious that if a person is having insufficient sleep, the intake of food will be increased. In addition, because of this there will be an increase in the weight of the person. The satisfaction after eating increases due to sleep deprivation. According to some epidemiological studies, it is also concluded that the people who sleep less are more obese as compared to those who have full-time sleep. Sleep deprivation is also a major causal factor of the increase in risk of developing type 2 diabetes. When the body is in the state of insufficient sleep, insulin resistance is more pronounced within the body's cells and hence the proper management of blood sugar is derailed.

Sleep loss and the Immune System:

Sleep is a natural defense mechanism to protect our body from infections. It enhances the immune system and allows it to function with full capability when dealing with diseases and viruses. A lack of sleep would undoubtedly throw a spanner in the works. It was found that people who sleep less were more at risk of catching the common cold and other infectious ailments.

Cancer has also been linked to sleep loss, where studies have shown that tumor growth are amplified with the lack of sleep due to adjustments in production of tumor associated macrophages. Proper sleep seems to boost the production of tumor inhibiting macrophages, while the converse was true when it came to sleep deprivation. The consistent inflammation due to the overactive sympathetic nervous system brought on by lack of sleep is also considered to be one of the cancer promoting factors.

Sleep loss, Genes, and DNA

Sleep loss is the major reason for increased chances of Alzheimer's diseases, diabetes, heart diseases, obesity, depression, hypertension, and other fatal diseases. It affects the functioning of DNA also and weakens the memory circuits of your brain. Almost all the proper functioning of the brain depends on having proper sleep.

Chapter 9 -
Sleep & Dreams

Key Knowledge Pointers

- MRI scans can detect brain activity in specific regions of the brain during REM sleep.

- During REM sleep, some portions of the brain are 30% more active than they are during the wakeful state.

- The visuospatial regions, motor cortex, amygdala, and cingulate cortex, and hippocampus are more active during the REM stage.

- Ancient Egyptians and Greeks believed that dreams are sent down from the gods. Aristotle believed that dreams stem from the events during our waking time.

- 35-55% of the emotions an individual experiences while awake also resurface during dreams.

MRI (Magnetic resonance imaging) scans can detect brain activity in specific portions of the brain. During NREM sleep, the metabolic activity level drops. However, during the dream REM sleep, the metabolic activity in the brain rises. This increase in activity is identified in four major areas: visuospatial regions, motor cortex, amygdala and cingulate cortex, and hippocampus. In REM sleep, there is a 30% rise in activity in these areas as compared to wake state.

Moreover, the regions of the prefrontal cortex experience a decrease in brain activity levels during REM sleep. The prefrontal cortex is the decision-maker and logical thinker of our brains.

So, during REM sleep, our cognitive abilities decrease, while the motor, emotion and autobiographical memory areas of the brain are activated.

Thanks to MRI, it is possible to predict the form of an individua's dream. So, a researcher can accurately predict whether the dream is emotional, motor, or visual.

Dr. Yukiyasu Kamitani also managed to find the content of dreams using MRI. It was just like the researchers could mind read the participants of the research study. So, through such methods, it is possible to help disorders that involve issues with dreams.

This also leads to potential ethical concerns if this method becomes widespread and more efficient in the future.

The Meaning of Dreams

MRI scans have helped to understand the form of dreams. However, the question remains: where do dreams actually come from?

Ancient Egyptians and Greeks believed that dreams are sent down from the gods. Aristotle believed that dreams stem from the events during our waking time.

Sigmund Freud believed that dreams gave their origins in the brain and unconscious wishes. He defined the latent and manifest content of dreams. He offered generic dream interpretations. However, his interpretations were not reliable and consistent. Some of them were generic and seemed to fit anyone's dreams regardless of personal differences.

Today, brain scans claim that dreams arise from our own experiences as the autobiographical regions of the brain are very active during REM sleep.

However, Stickgold conducted research to verify this and found that only 1-2% of the dream content stemmed from 'day residue.'

Another discovery was that 35-55% of the emotions an individual experiences while awake also resurface during dreams.

Chapter 10 -
Therapy Through Overnight Dreams

Key Knowledge Pointers

- Researchers used to believe that dreaming is an epiphenomenon of REM sleep and doesn't offer any major benefits.

- It is possible that REM sleep is the only time in the entire day when your brain doesn't supply noradrenaline.

- REM sleep and dreams during it can help to recall important experiences without feeling the pain associated with the experiences.

- The high levels of noradrenaline in PTSD patients lead to a disturbance from entering the normal REM sleep.

- Depriving an individual of REM sleep also decreases their ability to pinpoint the differences between subtle nuances in facial expressions.

Researchers have long believed that dreams are just an epiphenomenon or by-product of REM sleep. They believed that dreaming doesn't have any benefits of its own.

It was thought that evolution accidentally created dreaming while it was constructing the neural pathways of the brain.

However, this is far from the truth. There are two benefits of REM sleep and dreams. First, they both help our emotional and mental health and rejuvenates our emotional resolution. Secondly, dreams and REM sleep are essential for problem solving and creativity.

Dream Therapy

REM sleep and dreaming can help you recover from painful and traumatic emotional experiences. They can take the pain away from traumatic experiences so that you can remember the event without having to relive the entire emotions as well. So, the next morning you wake up after a quality REM sleep night with dreams, your emotions will feel more resilient than before.

During the REM sleep period, our brain shuts off the supply of noradrenaline or the stress hormone. It is possible that REM sleep is the only time in the entire day when your brain doesn't supply noradrenaline.

It is known that the emotion and memory-related portions are active during the time of dreaming and REM sleeps. The amygdala and hippocampus are the specific areas that show a good amount of brain activity even during the time we are sleeping in the REM stage.

So, the emotional memories are active during REM sleep while the stress hormone level is zero. During REM sleep, the brain works on painful memories and experiences without the anxiety-triggering hormones in action.

It is then possible that REM sleep and dreams remove the intensity of pain from a traumatizing experience. This is the theory of overnight therapy.

It seems that REM sleep and dreams have two basic benefits:

1. Sleeping helps to consolidate memories so that we can remember them.
2. Sleeping also helps to forget the negative emotions and pain attached to experiences.

If you think back to an experience that traumatized you in the past, it might not have the same emotional effect again. You might still remember it precisely, but without reliving the emotional pain attached with that.

So, REM sleep and dreams during it can help to recall important experiences without feeling the pain associated with the experiences.

Imagine if we didn't have the benefit of REM sleep. We would be anxious all the time!

A study was conducted on a group of healthy adults. The participants were shown images and they rated how emotional they felt.

Then, half of the participants viewed the images again in the evening, having been awake all day. The other half viewed the images after sleeping.

The group that slept reported fewer emotions when they saw the images again. Their MRI scans also reported a decrease in the activity in the amygdala.

This shows that sleep decreased the emotions they attached with the same experience.

Dr. Rosalind Cartwright studied the dreams of the people who were going through depression. He noticed that these people had the same emotional themes in their dreams.

He also observed that the patients who dream about the painful experiences resolved them and had no depression later. However, the individuals who were dreaming, but not about the painful experiences suffered from depression due to them.

So, it seemed that REM sleep with general dreams alone does not help to resolve such emotional experiences. REM sleep along with dreams about the specific experiences leads to clinical remission.

The patients with PTSD suffered from trauma when they had not gone over the experiences in their dreams. The high levels of noradrenaline in PTSD patients lead to a disturbance from entering the normal REM sleep.

If their levels of noradrenaline could be lowered, they would be able to get rid of the strong emotions attached to the trauma. A drug called prazosin helped to decrease the levels of noradrenaline in the brain, leading to a better REM sleep quality.

Depriving an individual of REM sleep also decreases their ability to pinpoint the differences between subtle nuances in facial expressions.

Chapter 11 -
Creativity & Control with
Dreaming

Key Knowledge Pointers

- NREM sleep consolidates individual memories, while REM sleep interconnects these memories in new ways that promote abstract thought.

- Dreaming has some amazing creative functions that many great people have harnessed REM sleep and dreams during it can help to recall important experiences without feeling the pain associated with the experiences.

- REM sleep is also observed in language learning in infants.

- The content of dreams is also important for problem-solving.

- About 20% of the population is known to control their dreams, a phenomenon known as dream lucidity.

NREM sleep consolidates individual memories. On the other hand, REM sleep interconnects these memories in new ways that promote abstract thought.

For example, Dmitri Mendeleev had a dream that led to the creation of the periodic table. He had been working on the logic behind elements and couldn't arrive at any solution. After having been awake for three days, he went to sleep and had a dream.

Similarly, Otto Loewi discovered the role of neurotransmitters in firing electrical signals while he was sleeping. Paul McCartney created two of his amazing songs, "Yesterday" and "Let It Be" while he was dreaming.

So, it is obvious that dreaming has some amazing creative functions that many great people have harnessed. However, just the evidence that these people have used dreaming to their benefit doesn't provide a scientific study.

To prove this scientifically a study was conducted by the author and Stickgold. They used the sleep inertia period to give a ninety-seconds test to the participants. The participants were given a task that required creativity to solve. For example, they were presented with a puzzle to solve.

After the sleep inertia phase from NREM sleep, the participants didn't seem to be very creative on the tasks. However, when they were woken out of REM sleep, their creativity levels had increased.

The effect of the REM sleep of semantic knowledge was also tested. When the brain wakes up from NREM sleep, it builds logical relationships between concepts. However, when the brain wakes up from REM sleep, it creates links that are new and creative. It seems that during REM sleep, the brain is inclined towards finding novel solutions rather than the common sense ones.

Dr. Jeffret Ellenbogen tested the phenomenon of connectedness. REM sleep helped to establish distant and unique connections between memories even though the connections were not suggested while the individual was awake.

So, studies on the magics of REM sleep show that REM sleep helps to increase wisdom and comprehension as opposed to simple knowledge and learning.

REM sleep can create abstract and complex concepts by linking together past and present memories.

REM sleep is also observed in language learning in infants. It helps to make grammatical rules more abstract and interconnected, thereby helping with language skills.

The content of dreams is also important for problem-solving. If an individual doesn't dream about content related to the subject at hand, dreams don't have the same effect of aiding in creativity and problem-solving.

Robert Stickgold conducted an experiment to test this phenomenon. He used a virtual maze and placed some visual cues in it to help the individual find his way through it.

Then, half of the group slept for ninety minutes while the other half stayed awake. The group that went to sleep were awakened briefly in the middle of REM sleep to ask about the content of their dreams.

Among the group that slept and had dreams related to content showed ten times more improvement in performance as compared to the other two groups.

So, it seems that sleep and dreams don't simply recreate an individual's experiences but rather they attempt to piece together knowledge by making complex linkages among new and pre-existing memories.

Controlling your Dreams

About 20% of the population is known to control their dreams, a phenomenon known as dream lucidity.

During REM sleep, all muscles, except for the eye muscles are paralyzed. So, a study was conducted to test out this subjective experience of controlling dreams. The participants would signal to the researchers through eye movements to let them know that they were moving their hands in the dream. MRI scans detected brain activity as if the individual was actually moving their hands.

So, this provided objective evidence that lucid dreamers can control their dreams.

Chapter 12 -
Sleep Problems & Disorders

Key Knowledge Pointers

- Somnambulism refers to sleep (somnus) disorders in which the individual shows some kind of movement (ambulation)

- Insomnia is the most common sleep disorder.

- About one in 2000 people suffers from the neurological disorder known as narcolepsy.

- Fatal Familial Insomnia (FFI) is a rare sleep disorder in which the patient can't sleep.

Somnambulism

Somnambulism refers to sleep (somnus) disorders in which the individual shows some kind of movement (ambulation) such as sleep talking, sleepwalking, sleep sex, homicide, etc.

The movement occurs in the deep NREM sleep when the individual is neither awake nor asleep. Brain activity will show that the person is deep asleep with the brain waves of NREM sleep while the person is doing something and looks awake.

Mostly, sleepwalking and talking is not harmful and don't need treatment. It is more common in children than adults as children spend more time in NREM sleep. However, if sleepwalking poses a health risk, medical attention is necessary.

Insomnia

Insomnia is the most common sleep disorder. It involves an inability to sleep even though the individual tries to sleep. It is different from sleep deprivation.

There are two forms of insomnia: onset insomnia in which the person has difficulty falling asleep and maintenance insomnia in which the person finds it hard to stay asleep. Both the forms may occur together, or separately. The diagnostic criteria include daytime dysfunction and having insomnia for at least three nights for every week up to three months for a sleep disturbance to qualify for insomnia. Despite such thorough criteria, it is one of the most common sleep disorders in many adults.

Insomnia is twice as common in women than in men. If you have trouble sleeping, you should go to a sleep doctor instead of your GP to get a thorough diagnosis and appropriate treatment if required.

The most common causes of insomnia are psychological and emotional such as anxieties, overthinking, etc. Patients have a higher heart rate due to noradrenaline in their body and have trouble in reducing their core body temperature.

Narcolepsy

Narcolepsy occurs due to gene mutations but it is not inheritable. It is characterized by the following symptoms:

1. Extreme sleepiness during the day
2. Sleep paralysis
3. Cataplexy

About one in 2000 people suffers from this neurological disorder. Sleep paralysis is like becoming locked in one's own body immediately after waking up. It occurs after waking from REM sleep. One in four people will experience this symptom sometimes in their lives. However, in narcoleptics, it is extremely common. So, it is a symptom of narcolepsy but not exclusive to it.

Cataplectic attacks are triggered by extreme emotions, positive or negative. The individual experiences a seizure and falls, appearing to be unconscious. However, patients are awake during this and know what is going on around them. The muscle tone decreases and the body just collapses.

Any extreme emotion, happiness or sadness can cause this. So, these individuals are forced to live an emotionless life.

Narcoleptics have a decreased amount of the neurotransmitter orexin and its receptors. Orexin is essential for switching the sleep-wake switch in the hypothalamus.

There is no cure for this disease due to its rarity and a consequential lack of ample research to develop and test treatment. Common ways to deal with it include giving amphetamine or Provigil to fight against daytime sleepiness.

Fatal Familial Insomnia (FFI)

This is a rare sleep disorder in which the patient can't sleep. It has many consequences including a decline of cognitive abilities, organs are affected, hallucinations and delusions become common to the extent that the patient loses energy to walk and even talk.

It has no treatment and the patients are known to die within ten months or lesser of diagnosis.

The cause of this disorder is thought to be due to a prion protein gene PrNP that becomes anomalous. The sensory information cannot pass through the thalamus as it becomes damaged with holes.

Current treatment options include an antibiotic called doxycycline that can reduce the accumulation of the protein that causes this disorder.

Chapter 13 - Sleep Obstacles

Key Knowledge Pointers

- Exposure to light during the night time leads to a decrease in sleep quality.

- Alcohol can have two other drastic effects on sleep.

- If our brain regularly loses REM sleep, it starts to build up. If those go on for long, the individual will start to experience dreaming while they are awake. This leads to hallucinations, delusions and disorientation. This psychotic state is known as "delirium tremens."

"Sleep procrastination" is caused by many factors including the following:

1. Exposure to constant electric light
2. Regularized temperatures
3. Caffeine
4. Alcohol
5. Punching time cards

Exposure to Constant Electrical Light

After Thomas Edison built the power station, mankind started to control sleep and wake stages. Exposure to light during the night time leads to a decrease in sleep quality.

When the fire came into existence, humans started to use fire as a light to work during the dark. When gas and oil-burning lamps came, entire cities would be awake even during the night time. This led to an increase in waking up during the night.

However, when electric light bulbs were invented, our suprachiasmatic nucleus suffered the most. Normal sunlight contains all wavelengths of the visible spectrum: shorter wavelengths that look blue and violet, as well as longer wavelengths that are of red and yellow shades.

When the sunlight fades, our suprachiasmatic nucleus automatically knows that it is time to sleep. The pineal gland starts to release melatonin to help us fall asleep.

However, electric light canceled this neat order. Our brains no longer get the signal of darkness. So, our suprachiasmatic nucleus is fooled into thinking that it is still daytime.

By halting the natural release of melatonin due to exposure to artificial light before bedtime, makes it more likely that we will fall asleep later.

Furthermore, bedside lamps can also influence the natural patterns of the suprachiasmatic nucleus. Even dim light from the bedside lamp can delay the release of melatonin.

The dimmest bedside lamp gives a light of 20 to 80 lux, about 1-2% of the intensity from sunlight. Despite this, such lighting can have up to 50% suppression of natural melatonin release.

If things weren't already worst, the blue light from LEDs or light-emitting diodes has a twice as harmful impact on our melatonin levels.

Even if the intensities of blue light are the same as warm yellow light, blue wavelengths have the worst effect on melatonin levels.

Furthermore, the screens of our smartphones, laptops, and tablets emit blue light. A survey found that 90% of the individuals use an electronic device during the hour before going to bed.

A recent study found that using an iPad two hours prior to going to bed can actually reduce the melatonin levels by 23%.

Another recent study made a more interesting finding. The study included healthy adults for a two-week period. The adults were divided into two groups.

The first group was allowed to read a printed book before going to bed. They were not allowed to use any electronic devices. The second group could read a book on their iPad.

When both the groups were compared, it was observed that the iPad group suffered from a decrease in melatonin levels by 50% as compared to the other group. Moreover, they could fall asleep only in the early morning hours instead of the normal time. Also, it took them longer to fall asleep after being exposed to blue light from the iPad screen.

Exposure to blue light at night also altered the quality and quantity of their sleep. First, the amount of REM sleep decreased during the night. Second, they felt sleepy during the next day. Third, they experienced a ninety-minute delay in melatonin release for the next few days following the study even though they were not using the iPad at night in those days.

So, LED lights not only influence when we will fall asleep, but also how well we will sleep, how rested we will feel during the following day and the time of release of melatonin for the next few days.

Granted that the iPads and other electronic devices have many benefits, but they have the worst possible effects on our sleep that we need for the development of our brains. So, there are some ways to go about this and reduce the damage of electronic devices.

For example, it is possible to dim the light of the house an hour before bedtime. Some people even wear yellow-tinted glasses to screen the blue wavelengths that delay the release of melatonin.

You can also install software on your electronic devices to block out the blue wavelengths they emit. It is equally important to maintain complete darkness during the night.

Alcohol

It is a common myth that people sleep better due to alcohol. Alcohol is a sedative that prevents the neurons from sending chemicals through the brain. However, even though alcohol is a sedative, it can make you feel high.

The reason behind this is that alcohol sedates the prefrontal cortex of our brains. The frontal lobe is like the CEO of the brain that helps to control our behavior and impulses.

So, when alcohol sedates the frontal lobe region, we can "loosen up" and become less controlled. When alcohol sedates other parts of the brain, it makes us feel sluggish. We want to let go of our conscious state and fall into sedation. However, sedation is not equivalent to sleep.

So, alcohol may sedate you, but can't make you fall asleep. It seems that the state of sedation is like that of a light dose of anesthesia.

Moreover, alcohol can have two other drastic effects on sleep. First, alcohol will fragment sleep. So, you will wake up in the middle of the night several times. However, you may not remember waking up the next morning.

Many people relate alcohol to better sleep and don't realize that it makes them feel tired the next day.

Alcohol also affects the quantity of REM sleep. When the body breaks down alcohol, we get aldehydes and ketones that block the brain's ability to produce REM sleep. So, even a moderate amount of alcohol can deprive your brain of the much-needed dream sleep.

If our brain regularly loses REM sleep, it starts to buildup. If those go on for long, the individual will start to experience dreaming while they are awake. This leads to hallucinations, delusions and disorientation. This psychotic state is known as "delirium tremens."

If an alcohol addict goes to a rehabilitation center, the brain will go through a REM-sleep rebound.

REM sleep is essential for memory integration. So, researchers conducted a study on this. College participants learned a new type of grammar. Then, a week later, their retention was tested.

The first group of participants slept naturally. The second group of students drank a little before bedtime. In the third group, the participants slept naturally for the first and second nights and drunk on the third night.

On the seventh day, they were tested while sober. The first group showed excellent retention of knowledge and even showed abstract learning. On the other hand, the second group suffered from partial amnesia and forgot more than 50% of the content.

The third group also suffered from about 40% forgetting even though they had slept for the first and second night after learning. So, it seems that memories are vulnerable to disruption of sleep on even the third night.

Temperature

To fall asleep successfully, our core body temperature needs to drop by 1-2 degrees Fahrenheit. When the temperature falls, our suprachiasmatic nucleus starts to release melatonin.

So, temperature and light synergistically work together to release melatonin. Your hands, feet, and head become warmer so that the core temperature is a little lower.

A bedroom temperature of 65 degrees Fahrenheit is the best to fall asleep easily. Sleep clinicians have noticed that older adults sleep 18% faster with thermal assistance and insomniacs sleep 25% faster.

Hot baths before sleeping are known to induce deeper NREM sleep by 10-15% in healthy adults.

Alarms

When you are pulled away from your sleep by an alarm clock, your heart rate, and blood pressure increase due to the shock on the heart. When we snooze the alarm repeatedly, we alarm our hearts multiple times in a short period of time.

Chapter 14 -
Right & Wrong Sleeping Aids

Key Knowledge Pointers

- There are no drugs that can induce natural sleep.

- Sleeping pills have a more perceived benefit than they may actually do.

- Many non-pharmacological methods to treat insomnia including electrical and auditory stimulation methods, cognitive behavioral therapy are being used to replace sleeping pills to help insomniacs.

There are no drugs that can induce natural sleep. Even sleeping pills don't imitate the brain activity that is present during natural sleep.

Most sleeping pills will sedate your brain cortex rather than putting you to the deep-wave natural sleep. The electrical quality in sleep due to medication is deficient.

Furthermore, sleeping pills can create a vicious cycle that is very harmful in the long term. Sleeping pills can make you feel groggy the following day. As a result of that, you will opt for caffeinated drinks such as tea and coffee throughout the day. In turn, the caffeine will keep you awake at night, prompting you to take a sleeping pill. The cycle will repeat the next day, and so on.

What's worst is that you will develop a dependency on sleeping pills. If you don't take them, you will suffer from rebound insomnia due to withdrawal effects. You will also develop drug tolerance as sleeping pills are addictive.

Furthermore, sleeping pills have a more perceived benefit than they may actually do. Studies show that the difference between placebo and sleeping pills is not very significant. In both cases, the individual will fall asleep faster. It's ironic that this benefit is more subjective rather than objective.

A study reported that there are only slight improvements in sleep with sleeping pills. When these improvements are weighed against the long list of side effects, they are not worth it.

For example, we know that natural sleep helps to consolidate memories. However, sleeping pill induced sleep doesn't solidify memories in the same way. The story doesn't finish there. Sleeping pills also weaken previous memories. The average age of insomnia patients is also decreasing. So, sleeping pills are making the young generation forgetful.

So, they may help you fall asleep a little faster, but have other major concerns that cannot be ignored.

Dr. Daniel Kripke from the University of California found that sleeping pills may leave you more susceptible to cancer. There is a clear relationship between decreased mortality and sleeping pills. Those who take sleep medication are 4.6 times more likely to die over the next few years as compared to people who don't use such medicines. The statistics also vary with the frequency of usage.

A reason of this is attributed to the fact that natural sleep helps the body fight infections and build immunity. What's worst is that the older generation that is documented to be 50% of the sleep medication users are more susceptible to infections. When both the aspects work synergistically, though independently, they decrease mortality rates further.

It is also possible that decreased mortality due to sleeping pills may be related to road accidents due to grogginess while driving. We all know that sleep medications can cause grogginess the following day.

Summing up, it is also likely that the individuals who opt for sleep medication were already prone to health issues because of a lack of good sleep.

Substituting Sleeping Pills

Many non-pharmacological methods are being used to replace sleeping pills to help insomniacs. They include electrical and auditory stimulation methods, cognitive behavioral therapy for insomnia among many others.

Cognitive-behavioral therapy for insomnia or CBT-I addresses bad habits that lead to poor sleeping patterns. For example, if the patient suffers from anxiety and overthinking when they go to bed, this therapy tries to address the root issues that underlie these problems. Some instances of the therapy at work would be that the patients are suggested to spend the least amount of time on the bed. They should go to bed when they are tired and ready to sleep.

Cutting down on caffeine and alcohol, making regular bedtime routines, waking up and sleeping at the same times can help individuals to sleep better. They should avoid napping during the day and have a cool bedroom instead of a temperature-regulated one.

Chapter 15 -
Why We Should All Care

Key Knowledge Pointers

- Sleep deprivation negatively affects job performance, productivity, creativity and so many other domains that are essential for the workplace.

- Chronic sleep deprivation in adolescents can lead to chronic mental illnesses.

- Studies claim that medical residents who work for long shifts make 36% more mistakes that can lead to serious repercussions for the patients.

A century ago, just 2% of the US population slept for less than six hours a night. Today, nearly 30% of the people sleep for six hours and lesser. A 2013 survey found that more than 65% of the adults don't sleep the recommended eight hours.

Furthermore, it's not that these individuals don't want to sleep. On the weekends, they sleep more than eight hours in an attempt to make up for the lost sleep. However, it is not possible to "make up" for lost sleep. What's lost is lost.

So, you might think why should anyone beyond an individual care about sleep? This chapter addresses this question.

Sleep in the Workplace

Sleep deprivation is very common in the workplace. What's ironic is that no one cares about it. Sleep deprivation negatively affects job performance, productivity, creativity and so many other domains that are essential for the workplace. Even though all workplaces have strict policies against smoking, substance abuse, work ethics, etc. they don't care about the side effects of sleep deprivation.

People who sleep less at night cost a lot to their workplace due to the common errors attributed to sleep deprivation. Sleeping less affects the speed of work. It will take more time to do the same task when you are sleep deprived. I am not even talking about the accuracy of doing the task yet.

Also, people who sleep less don't like to take on challenging tasks. Moreover, businesses run on creativity. Sleep-deprived people are less creative. So, overworking people leads to loss rather than any benefit for the business.

Sleep deprivation also has effects on the individual's ethical behavior. Studies have observed that sleep-deprived people tend to show deviant behavior and lie more the following day. They will try to blame others for their own mistakes and also try to take the credit of other peoples' work.

Sleep deprivation is also linked to another phenomenon known as social loafing. This refers to people who like to participate in group activities so that they don't have to do a lot of work themselves.

Sleep-deprived CEOs and supervisors abuse their employees by being rude and disrespectful. They lose their self-control more often. This leads to the employees becoming less engaged in their jobs as well. So, it leads to a chain reaction whereby the supervisor's lack of sleep is affecting the entire team.

Sleep and Education

Teenagers and children must wake up very early for school. Remember that the circadian rhythm of teenagers shifts forward by one to three hours. Despite this, they have to wake up early and are expected to perform well in school.

Adolescents are susceptible to the development of many psychiatric illnesses such as schizophrenia, anxiety, and depression. So, chronic sleep deprivation in this age can lead to chronic mental illnesses.

A study was conducted in the 1960s. The participants were allowed to complete their NREM sleep but were deprived of REM sleep. As soon as they were about to fall in REM sleep, the researcher would wake them up. Then, they had to solve some mathematical problems so that they would not fall back asleep. Deprivation of REM sleep made them anxious, moody, and paranoid. They even started to get hallucinations. So, REM sleep is the difference between psychological wellness and mental illnesses.

Depriving teenagers and adolescents of late morning REM sleep due to early school time can lead to serious mental issues.

Identical twin studies also confirmed that sleep is a powerful factor that can even change the effect of genetic determinism.

Furthermore, the leading cause of death in students are road accidents. Sleep deprivation also plays a role in this.

A more interesting finding is that sleep deprivation in children is diagnosed as ADHD due to the similarity of the symptoms of both. What's more ironic is that the medications for ADHD, Adderall and Ritalin prevent the child's brain from sleeping. When the two add up, the symptoms aggravate and lead to more issues in children.

Recent surveys observed that more than 50% of children who have ADHD diagnosis are actually sleep-deprived.

Sleep Deprivation and Healthcare

We all know that medical residents are required to work for long hours without the luxury of sleep. The medical community believes that residents cannot learn the sheer amount of medical knowledge without putting in that time at the beginning of their career.

Halsted who introduced this concept was a cocaine addict. So, he could miraculously go without sleep for days without any problems.

Studies claim that residents who work for long shifts make 36% more mistakes that can lead to serious repercussions for the patients. Medical errors are the third most prevalent cause of death in the US after cancer and heart disease.

What's worst is that these sleep-deprived doctors get into fatal road accidents due to lack of sleep or commit suicide.

Many surgeons believe that they have "mastered" the art of sleeping lesser every day. However, this is not possible. You can't get used to ignoring sleep when Nature has spent millions of years to evolve it in its perfect form.

Chapter 16 –
New Views To Embrace Sleep

Key Knowledge Pointers

- We must understand the repercussions of lack of sleep and why this problem is hard to address.

- Educating people about the dangers that come with lack of sleep is vital, but it is not a solution in itself.

- Organizations should create policies for rewarding employees with incentives on the basis of sleep quality.

- Developing good sleep patterns as a society will have far-flung effects from reduced road accidents due to drowsiness, to decreased costs of medical issues that arise due to lack of sleep.

Now that we have talked about the problems caused by lack of sleep, let's talk about some solutions. First, we must understand the repercussions of lack of sleep and why this problem is hard to address.

Second, it is essential that we develop a strategy to deal with this issue systematically. There are multiple levels to fight the disease of lack of sleep.

1. Individual
2. Educational/ Interpersonal

3. Organizational
4. Public Policy/ Government
5. Societal

Let's discuss each of these one by one.

Individual Transformation

There are two kinds of methods to address sleep at a personal level. First, passive methods that require minimal effort from the individual. For example, installing smart thermostats to synchronize the environment's temperature with the natural drop in core temperature near bedtime. Another passive method is to decrease our exposure to blue wavelengths from light bulbs. We know that blue light dramatically affects the release of melatonin. On the other hand, using blue light in the mornings can make you feel more alert and active as it suppresses all the effects of melatonin.

This idea is used in spacecraft by NASA to give astronauts a regular pattern that imitates the twenty-four-hour day.

Educating people about the dangers that come with lack of sleep is vital, but it is not a solution in itself. We know the dangers of using digital devices before sleeping, but we still use them. So, it is essential that we convert this knowledge into actionable habits that become a way of life.

For example, apps that track your sleep data can help you identify deficits even when you don't realize it yourself. An app to discourage smoking modifies an individual's facial features to imitate the negative effects of smoking that will become visible in the near future if they continue their addiction.

Another essential aspect of proper sleep is immunity. Sleep is not only vital for the development of natural immunity, but also for artificial immunity. Flu shots are known to be more effective if you have been sleeping well during the week before. So, applications can help you determine the best time for flu shots. Working on sleep schedules can help to instill prevention over cure.

Educational Change

Everyone is educated on the benefits of a balanced diet, exercise and so on. However, education systems all over the world don't give sleep the attention it deserves.

By creating awareness about sleep, schools can help to create good sleep habits right from the beginning.

Organizational Change

Organizations should create policies for rewarding employees with incentives on the basis of sleep quality and duration by collecting their data through reliable sleep-tracking software.

This can have multi-fold benefits for both the organization and employees. The organization will benefit from productive, creative, happier employees who will be more willing to work. They will reduce the cost of employees going on sick leave or becoming less productive due to lack of sleep.

On the other hand, employees will gain a better health, longer life expectancy and overall satisfaction in life. Also, incentives, whether they are monetary or days off, will lead to more work satisfaction.

Organizations can also accommodate employees by creating different work slots for different chronotypes. Morning larks and night owls can work according to their comfort with flexible schedules. Both groups can have a common time slot that can be used for collaborative meetings. The benefits of this will extend beyond the organization and employees. For example, rush-hour traffic can be controlled efficiently.

Medical Sector

Sleep is also important for patients as well as residents in the medical sector. Studies claim that decreased quality or duration of sleep will make you more sensitive to pain along with other health issues.

Sleep is a natural analgesic that medical health professionals don't prescribe. It is free, readily available and a much better alternative to morphine. Morphine can have life-threatening side effects including breathing issues, as well as withdrawal symptoms, cold sweats, nausea, loss of appetite, etc. Moreover, morphine even prevents natural sleep.

So, sleep doesn't carry any of these side effects and also helps to improve our immune system to fight future infections.

Developing good sleep patterns as a society will have far-flung effects from reduced road accidents due to drowsiness, to decreased costs of medical issues that arise due to lack of sleep.

Conclusion

The human civilisation's descent into bucking the need for much needed sleep has been swift and decisive, and it happened all within 100 years. As a result, far reaching negative consequences are seen in our health, productivity as well as physical safety.

It is indeed time for us as a society to look at sleep for what it really is; an essential and important component that regulates our physiological as well as emotional health. The way we work and study needs to change in order to reflect this rediscovered importance of sleep in order for us to really reap the benefits.